TRIGGER POINT THERAPY

A Comprehensive Guide To Trigger Point Therapy: Discovering The Key To Pain-Free Living

DEAN OTTO

Contents

Introductory

The primary objective of trigger point massage is the release of trigger points within the musculature.

Trigger points are localized regions of muscle tension and constriction that, when compressed, can induce pain and distress in various anatomical regions. Frequently, these sites are tender and may give the sensation of taut bands or knots within the muscle.

Targeted pressure and massage techniques are utilized to identify and release these trigger points in trigger point therapy. Initially, the pressure applied by the massage therapist to the trigger points may induce pain or distress; however, the intensity of the pressure is typically modified in accordance with the client's tolerance. The sustained pressure improves blood flow to the area and aids in the relaxation of the contracted muscles.

Trigger point massage is frequently employed to treat chronic pain, muscle tension, restricted range of motion, and other musculoskeletal conditions.

Releasing trigger points is thought to alleviate discomfort and improve overall muscle health. Depending on the requirements of the individual, this form of massage may be integrated into a more comprehensive therapeutic massage session or it may constitute the central emphasis of the treatment.

It is crucial to acknowledge that although trigger point massage can provide advantages for numerous individuals, it may not be appropriate for all.

Before undergoing massage therapy, individuals with particular medical conditions or injuries should counsel a healthcare professional to ensure that the practice is safe and suitable for their particular circumstances. In addition, it is critical to convey any concerns or areas of discomfort to the massage therapist throughout the session.

CHAPTER ONE
The Significance Of Trigger Point Treatment

There are numerous factors why trigger point therapy may be beneficial, but especially for those who are afflicted with musculoskeletal pain and tension. The subsequent points underscore the significance of trigger point therapy:

• Analgesia: Trigger points are anatomically linked to specific regions of distress and pain. The purpose of trigger point therapy is to alleviate discomfort by releasing these knots or tight bands in the muscles. Through the targeted targeting of the specific anatomical components that cause discomfort, individuals may potentially attain a reduction in their pain levels.

• Enhanced Range of Motion Muscles that are contracted and tense can restrict the mobility and range of motion of joints. Trigger point therapy facilitates muscle relaxation and tension release, which may result in enhanced flexibility and improved mobility.

• Muscle Relaxation: Trigger point therapy induces muscle relaxation through the application of sustained pressure. This is particularly advantageous for those who suffer from persistent muscle tension, rigidity, or spasms.

• Increased Circulation: Trigger point therapy has the potential to improve blood flow to the targeted regions through the release of muscle tension. By facilitating the delivery of nutrients and oxygen to the muscles, enhanced circulation promotes healing and decreases inflammation.

• Prevention of Chronic Pain Trigger points are frequently implicated in chronic pain conditions. By addressing these trigger points early in the therapeutic process, long-term musculoskeletal health can be preserved by preventing the onset or worsening of chronic pain conditions.

• Supplementary Treatment for a Range of Conditions: migraines, myofascial pain syndrome, and fibromyalgia are among the conditions that frequently benefit from trigger point therapy. By being incorporated into a more comprehensive treatment regimen, it can effectively target particular symptoms while also promoting overall wellness.

- Muscular tension and pain are frequently observed symptoms that are linked to stress. In addition to ameliorating physical symptoms, trigger point therapy has the potential to induce relaxation and tension reduction, thereby fostering an enhanced state of overall health.

- Tailored Intervention: Trigger point therapy facilitates a more precise and personalized strategy for attending to particular regions of concern. The treatment can be tailored to the specific requirements and preferences of each client by a competent therapist.

It is imperative to acknowledge that although trigger point therapy can offer substantial benefits to numerous individuals, its efficacy may differ considerably among individuals.

Furthermore, it is imperative to seek guidance from a certified massage therapist or qualified healthcare practitioner in order to ascertain the suitability of trigger point therapy in relation to your particular health condition and requirements.

Point Of Trigger Formation

Trigger points, alternatively referred to as myofascial trigger points or muscle knots, denote contracted regions of muscle fibers that give rise to localized discomfort, soreness, and occasionally referred pain.

There are numerous variables that can influence the formation of trigger points, and their precise mechanisms remain unknown. Nonetheless, it is hypothesized that the following factors may contribute to the formation of trigger points.

• The occurrence of trigger points can be attributed to excessive muscle use or repetitive tension on a specific muscle or group of muscles. This phenomenon frequently manifests in occupations or activities that demand extended periods of muscle contraction or repetitive motion.

• Muscle Trauma or Injury: Trigger points may develop as a consequence of acute muscle trauma or injury. Muscle strains, sprains, and direct impact injuries are all examples.

• Inadequate Posture: Extended durations of suboptimal posture, such as prolonged periods spent seated at a desk with flawed ergonomics, may potentially contribute to the onset of trigger points. Incorrect muscle postures can result in tension and imbalances in the muscles.

• Muscle Imbalances: Trigger point formation can be exacerbated by imbalances between opposing muscle groups, in which certain muscles are overactive and others are underactive. A variety of factors, including muscle atrophy, joint instability, and improper movement patterns, can contribute to this imbalance.

• The physical manifestation of emotional stress and tension in the muscles can result in trigger points developing and heightened muscle tension. A complex relationship exists between muscle tension and stress, which may contribute to the development of chronic pain conditions.

• Muscle Function Impairment and Nutrition: Insufficient hydration and substandard nutrition may contribute to the development of trigger points. Undernourished and dehydrated muscles may be more susceptible to experiencing rigidity and spasms.

• Referred pain occurs when trigger points are responsible for the discomfort felt in a region remote from the site of the trigger point. It is critical to comprehend these referred pain patterns in order to address trigger points effectively.

It is imperative to acknowledge that ongoing research continues to focus on the comprehension of trigger points and their development. Moreover, trigger points are highly variable among individuals; the underlying factors that induce them in one person may not necessarily be the same in another. Trigger point treatment typically combines a variety of techniques, such as manual therapy, massage, stretching, and occasionally medication.

It is recommended that individuals suffering from chronic or severe pain related to trigger points seek the assistance of a qualified therapist or healthcare professional for evaluation of their unique circumstances and provision of treatment recommendations.

CHAPTER TWO
Determination Of Trigger Points

The process of identifying trigger points can be intricate, frequently necessitating the collaboration of an experienced individual and, at times, a trained medical professional. General guidelines for identifying trigger points are as follows:

1. Palpation performed by an expert:

• Manual therapists, including chiropractors, massage therapists, and physical therapists, are skilled in the technique of trigger point identification via palpation. They feel for tight bands or knots in the muscles using their fingertips.

• Medical professionals, including doctors, may evaluate trigger points as part of a routine physical examination. They might inquire about pain patterns and identify tender areas through palpation.

2. Anxiety Patterns:

• Trigger points frequently elicit distinct patterns of pain or discomfort. Gaining an understanding of the referred pain patterns that are linked to trigger points can facilitate the determination of their precise location.

• Anxiety can manifest not only at the specific location of the trigger point but also in peripheral regions of the organism. Such a condition is referred pain.

3. The process of self-examination:

• On occasion, individuals may be able to discern trigger points by means of self-examination. This procedure entails performing a light fingertip palpation of muscles in order to detect any tenderness, constriction, or knots.

- Self-examination of deeper muscles may present a greater challenge than that of superficial muscles.

4. Visual and Functional Evaluation:

- Potential trigger points can be deduced through the observation of movement and posture patterns. Visual manifestations of muscle imbalances and regions of heightened tension are possible.

- Functional movement assessment can be utilized to detect regions characterized by limited range of motion or discomfort.

5. Concerning Tender Points:

• In many cases, trigger points are tender to the contact. One method of identifying tenderness is by applying gentle pressure to the suspected area.

• A specific point of tenderness may serve the dual purpose of signaling the existence of a trigger point and distinguishing it from alternative analgesic sources.

6. The patient's medical history:

• Gaining knowledge about the activities and medical history of a patient can offer valuable insights into the possible etiology of trigger points. Contributing factors may include repetitive motion, chronic tension, or trauma.

It is imperative to acknowledge that the process of identifying and evaluating trigger points can be intricate, with the potential for misdiagnosis.

Experts who have received specialized training in musculoskeletal assessment and manual therapy methods are most qualified to precisely identify and treat trigger points.

In the event that you suspect that trigger points are the source of your persistent pain or distress, you may wish to seek the advice of a licensed manual therapist or healthcare professional for a comprehensive assessment and suitable intervention.

The Scientific Basis For Trigger Points

Despite the fact that trigger points have been the subject of extensive scientific investigation, further research is required to fully comprehend the underlying mechanisms. The following are fundamental scientific principles underlying trigger points:

1. Cotraction of Muscle Fibers:

• Trigger points are hypothesized to consist of areas of skeletal muscle tense bands that are hyperirritable. These tense bands frequently have a palpable quality and can resemble knots.

• It is hypothesized that muscle fibers are contracted within these tense bands, which results in heightened muscle tension and the development of a localized trigger point.

2. Shifts in Metabolic Rate and Ischemia:

• Ischemia can result from the prolonged contraction of muscle fibers in trigger points, which can cause a reduction in blood flow to the affected region. This decreased blood flow could potentially be a factor in the accumulation of metabolic detritus.

- Ischemia and the buildup of substances such as lactic acid in trigger points potentially contribute to the sensation of pain and the distinctive tenderness that is commonly associated with these areas.

3. Endplate Motor Dysfunction:

- There are certain hypotheses that propose the involvement of motor endplate dysfunction, the site of communication between nerve and muscle fibers, in the development of trigger points.

- Causes of sustained muscle contraction and the formation of trigger points may include disturbances in the normal signaling between nerves and muscles.

4. Aspects of the Neurological System:

• Trigger points are characterized by heightened peripheral nerve sensitivity. Enhanced sensitivity of the nerves in and around trigger points to stimuli may exacerbate pain and discomfort.

• Additionally, the response of the nervous system to emotional and stress-related factors may contribute to the formation and persistence of trigger points.

5. Referred Phenomenon of Pain:

• Referred pain, which occurs when the pain is perceived in an area far from the trigger point itself, is one of the distinguishing characteristics of trigger points.

• Although the precise mechanism underlying referred pain remains unknown, it is hypothesized to be comprised of intricate neural pathways and the aggregation of sensory signals within the spinal cord.

6. Biomechanical Aspects:

• Inadequate posture, muscular imbalances, and repetitive stress are biomechanical factors that potentially contribute to the onset of trigger points.

• Trigger points can develop in the presence of imbalances among muscle groups, modifications in movement patterns, or excessive demand on specific muscles.

7. Environmental and Genetic Factors:

• The susceptibility of an individual to trigger points may be influenced by genetic factors, while environmental factors including trauma, injuries, or chronic stress may play a role in their development.

It is noteworthy that the comprehension of trigger points is undergoing a process of development, and distinct viewpoints regarding their underlying mechanisms may exist among healthcare professionals.

A combination of manual therapies, including trigger point release techniques and massage, and interventions that target underlying factors including tension, posture, and movement patterns are frequently incorporated into treatment strategies.

Ongoing investigations into the fundamental mechanisms of trigger points may in the future pave the way for more precise and efficacious therapeutic strategies.

CHAPTER THREE
Treatment Of Frequent Conditions With Trigger Point Massage

A trigger point massage is frequently incorporated into comprehensive treatment plans for a variety of musculoskeletal disorders.

It is crucial to acknowledge that massage therapy, encompassing trigger point massage, may not offer a panacea for specific ailments. However, it can serve as a beneficial element of a comprehensive treatment regimen, mitigating symptoms and enhancing general welfare.

The following are frequent conditions that trigger point massage is frequently used to treat:

1. Tension and Pain in Muscles:

• A common application of trigger point massage is to alleviate general muscle tension and discomfort. This can manifest in various anatomical regions, such as the back, shoulders, neck, and shoulders.

2. Migraines and Headaches:

• Muscle trigger points in the shoulder and neck are frequently linked to tension headaches and migraines. The application of trigger point techniques during massage therapy may alleviate headache symptoms.

3. Symptoms of Myofascial Pain Syndrome:

• Myofascial pain syndrome is characterized by the manifestation of trigger points in the fascia and muscles that surround them. Utilizing trigger point massage to alleviate pain and enhance function is a prevalent strategy among those afflicted with this condition.

4. The fibromyalgia condition:

• Chronic fibromyalgia is distinguished by its extensive

distribution of musculoskeletal pain. In some cases, trigger point massage is incorporated into the treatment regimen as a means of targeting particularized regions of pain and discomfort.

5. Injuries in Sports:

• Trigger point massage has the potential to assist athletes in rectifying muscle imbalances, alleviating tension, and expediting the recuperation process following sports-related injuries.

6. Chronic Pain Disorders:

• Specific pain locations associated with chronic pain, such as sciatica or chronic low back pain, may be alleviated through the application of trigger point massage.

7. Imbalances of Posture:

• Adverse body posture may be a factor in the onset of trigger points. Trigger point massage has the potential to alleviate discomfort, correct muscular imbalances, and enhance posture.

8. Disorder of the Temporomandibular Joint (TMJ):

• Muscle trigger points in the mandible may be a factor in TMJ dysfunction. By employing massage therapy, specifically intraoral massage techniques, tension in the mandible muscles may be alleviated.

9. Strain Repetitive Injuries:

• Trigger point massage may be advantageous for individuals who have sustained repetitive strain injuries, including but not limited to carpal tunnel syndrome and tennis elbow, as it can alleviate discomfort and alleviate muscle tension.

10. Tension Relating to Stress:

• Emotional tension and stress frequently materialize in the muscular system. A trigger point massage can aid in the release of tension, the alleviation of stress, and the enhancement of general health.

It is crucial to acknowledge that although trigger point massage can provide advantages for a considerable number of people, its suitability may not extend to all individuals and its efficacy may differ.

Healthcare personnel should be consulted by individuals with specific medical conditions or injuries in order to ascertain the safety and suitability of trigger point massage as an integral component of their comprehensive treatment regimen.

A comprehensive approach, which may also involve lifestyle modifications, exercises, and additional therapies, is frequently advised for the treatment of musculoskeletal disorders.

Implements And Methods Of Trigger Point Massage

In order to alleviate pain and distress, trigger point massage entails the application of pressure to particular areas of muscle tension and tightness.

In order to effectively target trigger points, massage therapists employ a variety of instruments and techniques. The following are frequent implements and methodologies utilized in trigger point massage:

The tools are:

1. Hands and Fingers:

• Trigger point massage is predominantly performed with the therapist's hands and fingertips. By applying direct pressure to the trigger points, they palpate the musculature for tight bands or knots.

2. Balls, knobs, or pressure instruments:

• Therapists may employ handheld instruments featuring knobs or spheres in order to exert pressure on trigger points. These instruments enable more sustained and concentrated pressure, which can be especially beneficial when performing deep tissue manipulation.

3. Rollers and Sticks for Massage:

• In order to target specific muscle areas, one may utilize massage rollers or poles featuring textured surfaces. Frequently, these implements are utilized in conjunction with therapist-assisted massage or for self-massage.

4. Cupping Treatment:

• Cupping is a technique that employs suction cups to induce negative pressure on the epidermis. By targeting particular trigger point areas, it facilitates blood circulation, alleviates tension, and mitigates discomfort.

5. Cold/Heated Therapy:

• Additionally, cold packs or heat cushions may be applied alongside trigger point massage. Cold therapy can decrease inflammation, whereas heat can aid in muscle relaxation.

The individual's condition and the characteristics of the trigger point will determine which method—warmth or cold—is utilized.

6. Percussion and Vibration Devices:

• Vibrating or percussion massage apparatus have the potential to effectively target trigger points. By applying rapid, repetitive motions to the muscle, these apparatuses aid in tension relief and enhance blood circulation.

Methods of Technique:

1. Static compression involves:

• Sustained, direct pressure is exerted on the site of activation. The pressure is maintained by the therapist until the muscle releases tension.

2. Deep striking or stripping:

• To loosen and extend constricted muscles, long, gliding strokes are executed along the muscle fibers. The integration of static compression with this technique can be applied to particular trigger points.

3. Fiber-to-Fiber Friction:

• By applying pressure perpendicular to the muscle fibers, the therapist facilitates the dissolution of adhesions and the release of tension in the trigger points.

4. The stretch:

• Stretching, whether passive or active, may be used in conjunction with trigger point therapy. Stretching reduces muscle tension and increases flexibility.

5. Massage of the Intraoral Space:

• When addressing trigger points in the facial muscles or jaw, clinicians may employ intraoral massage methods. This involves relaxing tension in the muscles within the pharynx.

6. Release of the Myofascial Tissue:

• Supplementing trigger point therapy with techniques that target the fascia, the connective tissue that envelops muscles, is a common practice. The process may entail applying sustained, moderate pressure in order to loosen fascial restrictions.

It is crucial to acknowledge that the selection of instruments and techniques, as well as the application of trigger point massage, are contingent upon the therapist's evaluation, the characteristics of the trigger points, and the particular requirements of the individual.

It is recommended that you seek guidance from a licensed massage therapist or healthcare professional in order to ascertain the most suitable method for managing trigger points in light of your specific circumstances.

Strengthening And Elongating Exercises

Incorporating stretching and strengthening exercises into a

comprehensive fitness and wellness regimen are fundamental elements. They improve mobility, flexibility, and the overall condition of the muscles.

Stretching and strengthening exercises for a variety of muscle groups are illustrated below. It is advisable to seek guidance from a healthcare professional prior to commencing any new exercise regimen, particularly if you have any pre-existing health conditions or concerns.

Stretching Performing:

1. Neck Expansion:

- Achieve a slight lateral tilt of the cranium while directing the ear toward the shoulder. After 15 to 30 seconds of holding, repeat on the opposite side.

2. Shoulder Expansion:

- Cross the right arm over the torso. Employing your left hand, deftly draw your right arm inward towards your torso. After 15 to 30 seconds of holding, alternate sides.

3. Triceps Expansion:

- Bend the elbow of your right arm while raising it overhead and extend your hand down your back. Apply a light pressure with your left hand on your right elbow. After 15 to 30 seconds of holding, alternate sides.

4. The chest opener is:

• Originate your limbs and clasp your hands behind your back. Raise your arms marginally and expand your thorax. Maintain for fifteen to thirty seconds.

5. Cat-Cow Stretch (Extension and Flexion of the Spine):

• To begin, place yourself on your hands and knees. Exhale while rounding your back (cat pose) and inhale while arching your back (cow pose). Continue for one to two minutes.

6. Fold Forward:

• Maintain a hip-width distance between your ankles and hinge at your hips while reaching toward the floor. In order to stretch the hamstrings and lower back, maintain for 15 to 30 seconds.

7. Flexor of the hip stretch:

• Perform a lunge by advancing your right foot while maintaining an extended left leg behind you. Engage in the stretch with your left hip flexor in motion. After 15 to 30 seconds of holding, alternate sides.

8. Quad Stretching Position:

• While standing on one leg, approach your buttocks with the opposite foot while grasping its ankle with your hand. After 15 to 30 seconds, switch legs.

9. The calf stretch:

• Position yourself with one foot forward and one foot back, facing a wall. While flexing the front knee, maintain a straight back leg. After 15 to 30 seconds, switch legs.

10. Forward Seated Bend:

• While seated, extend your legs in front of you. Aim toward your toes while articulating at your hips. Maintain for fifteen to thirty seconds.

Resistance-Building Exercises:

1. Weight-Bearing Squats:

• Proceed by maintaining a shoulder-width distance between your feet, squat back into a chair position, and subsequently rise to a standing stance.

2. Perform push-ups:

• To begin, assume a plank position and bend your elbows to lower your body toward the ground. Reestablish contact with the starting position by pushing upwards.

3. The plank:

- While in the plank position, align your body from your head to your heels in a straight line. Maintain contraction of your core muscles for thirty seconds to one minute.

4. As for lunges:

- Initiate the movement by advancing one foot forward while bending both knees at a 90-degree angle. After returning to the starting position, alternate legs.

5. Cross-Bent Rows:

- O-Hinge at your hips while holding a dumbbell in each hand and row the weights toward your chest while contracting your shoulder blades.

6. The bicep curl:

• While grasping a dumbbell in each hand, curl the weights toward one's shoulders while keeping the palms facing forward.

7. Diced Triceps:

• Position yourself at the periphery of a chair or bench, grasp your hands at your hips, and extend your body from the seat through arm straightening.

8. Lifting deadlifts:

• Maintaining a straight back, hinge at the hips and lower the weights toward the ground using a barbell or dumbbells. Recumb back to an upright position.

9. Leg raises:

• While lying on your back, extend your legs in a straight line toward the ceiling. Reposition them so that they do not make contact with the floor.

10. Diverse Plank Variations:

• Incorporate alternative exercises such as plank with leg lifts, side planks, and other variants to effectively target distinct muscle groups.

Warm up prior to performing any stretching exercises, and then gradually increase the difficulty of the strengthening routine. It is recommended that individuals with pre-existing health conditions or concerns consult a fitness professional or healthcare provider prior to commencing a new exercise regimen.

CHAPTER FOUR
Establishing A Session Of Trigger Point Massage

The development of a successful trigger point massage session necessitates meticulous preparation, attentiveness to the client's requirements, and adept execution of massage methodologies. A procedural outline for establishing a trigger point massage session is as follows:

1. Client Evaluation:

• Commence by conducting a comprehensive evaluation of the client's medical background, encompassing any concurrent ailments, injuries, or areas of apprehension.

• Inquire about the client's present symptoms, degree of pain, and objectives regarding the massage session.

2. The Art of Communication:

• Establish effective client communication. Outline their preferences, expectations, and any particular aspects that they would like the session to concentrate on.

• Encourage the client to communicate throughout the session regarding comfort and pressure levels, and inquire about their pain tolerance.

3. Postural Evaluation:

• Perform a postural evaluation in order to detect any muscular imbalances or regions of tension. Critical insights into potential trigger points can be obtained by observing the client's posture.

4. Target Setting:

• I will work in conjunction with the client to establish precise objectives for the session. The objectives might encompass relaxation, pain alleviation, or enhanced range of motion, among others.

5. Management Strategy:

• Incorporate trigger point massage techniques into a treatment plan formulated in accordance with the assessment results and the client's objectives.

• Determine precise trigger points that require attention and devise a methodical sequence of techniques to effectively target them.

6. In advance, preparation:

• Arrange a comfortable massage table, dim lighting, and soothing music in the massage room. Ensure the temperature of the room is suitable for habitation.

• Prepare any necessary equipment or tools, including massage oils, hot and cold packs, and specialized trigger point tools.

7. Client Placement:

• Provide the client with guidance regarding their proper positioning on the massage table. Offer suitable draping in order to guarantee both comfort and modesty.

• When positioning the client, ensure that the areas containing trigger points are easily accessible.

8. Manual Massage Methods:

• Employ a variety of trigger point massage techniques, such as stretching, deep stroking, cross-fiber friction, and static compression.

• Employ incremental pressure to trigger points while maintaining communication with the client to ascertain their comfort and making necessary adjustments to the pressure.

9. Implement Stretching:

• By incorporating stretching exercises into the session, the efficacy of trigger point therapy can be enhanced. This can assist in increasing muscular flexibility and relieving tension.

10. Reevaluation and Modifications:

• Reevaluate the client's response to the massage on a periodic basis. Solicit patient input regarding pain levels and modify the course of treatment accordingly.

• Adapt methodologies in accordance with the client's input and your own observations throughout the session.

11. At last:

• Towards the conclusion of the session, systematically transition by integrating more gentle massage strokes.

• Provide a summation of the session to the client, encompassing significant discoveries, advancements achieved, and suggestions for personal well-being.

12. After-Massage Suggestions:

• Offer post-massage suggestions, including but not limited to stretching exercises, hydration, and any other self-care routines that could further enhance the therapeutic effects of the session.

13. Sustained Action:

• Dialogue regarding the possible necessity for subsequent sessions in light of the client's progress and treatment objectives.

• Promote active client participation in communicating any ongoing concerns or changes to you.

Bear in mind that every client is distinct, and it is vital to customize the session according to their particular requirements. Constant communication with the client and adaptability in your approach are elements that contribute to the success of a trigger point massage session. Furthermore, maintain awareness of the most recent advancements in the field of massage therapy and further hone your abilities by participating in professional development activities.

Personal Care And Domestic Routines

The implementation of self-care and home practices is critical in sustaining the advantageous effects of trigger point massage and fostering holistic wellness. The following are some at-home self-care practices that individuals may implement:

1. Stretching Regimen:

• Consistently engage in stretching routines that concentrate on key muscle groups. Concentrate on trigger points or high-tension areas, including the shoulders, back, legs, hips, and shoulders.

2. The Foam Rolling Method:

• An foam roller can be employed to execute self-myofascial release. By rolling over various muscle groups, one can facilitate the release of tension, enhance flexibility, and decrease the probability of developing trigger points.

3. Cold and heat treatments:

• By utilizing warm compresses or heat packs, one can enhance blood circulation and muscle relaxation. Inflammation can be reduced with cold packs applied to areas experiencing acute pain or recent injury.

4. Utilizing Epsom Salt Baths:

• Soak in a warm bath containing Epsom salts to alleviate muscle soreness and promote relaxation. Magnesium is present in Epsom salts; it is soluble via the skin and has the potential to alleviate muscle tension.

5. Sufficient hydration:

• Maintain adequate hydration to promote muscle health as a whole. In addition to being vital for muscle function, water can aid in the elimination of toxins.

6. Respiratory Exercises:

• Engage in deep breathing exercises as a means to induce relaxation and alleviate stress. By utilizing the diaphragm, one can assist in the release of bodily tension.

7. Mental-Body Exercises:

• One should participate in mind-body exercises, such as tai chi or yoga, in order to enhance flexibility, balance, and mindfulness. These practices have the potential to enhance one's overall state of well-being.

8. Implementing Self-Massage Methods:

• One should acquire knowledge of and engage in the practice of self-massage techniques that target particular trigger points. Employ massage implements, your hands, fingers, or both, to apply pressure to areas of tension.

9. Developing Posture Awareness:

• Throughout the day, maintain proper posture, especially if you have a desk job. Consistently assess and rectify your posture in order to avert the development of trigger points and muscle imbalances.

10. Stress Administration:

• One should integrate stress management techniques, including relaxation exercises, mindfulness, and meditation, into their daily routine. Chronic stress may contribute to the development of trigger points and muscle tension.

11. Consistent Exercise:

• Regular physical activity reduces the risk of trigger points and maintains muscle health. Incorporate into your routine a variety of strengthening, flexibility, and cardiovascular exercises.

12. Sufficient Sleep:

- Ensure you are sleeping enough each night. Sleep quality is vitally important for both muscle recovery and general health.

13. Optimal Nutrition:

- It is essential to adhere to a well-balanced and nourishing diet in order to promote optimal muscle recovery and function. It is imperative to maintain a sufficient consumption of vitamins and minerals.

14. Consideratory Self-Reflection:

- It is imperative to be mindful of one's body and its signals. By engaging in consistent self-reflection, one can discern areas of stress, anxiety, or unease and proactively devise measures to remediate them.

15. Constructive Check-In:

- It is advisable to consult a healthcare professional, such as a physical therapist or massage therapist, for individualized treatment and advice if you are experiencing persistent or severe pain.

Customizing self-care practices to suit one's specific needs and preferences is of paramount importance. Incorporating these practices into your daily or weekly schedule can contribute to improved muscle health, decreased tension, and an enhanced sense of well-being; consistency is of the essence.

Summary

Trigger point massage represents a beneficial therapeutic modality in the management of muscular tension, pain, and discomfort. Trigger point science entails the detection and management of particular regions of muscle tension that are constricted, frequently accompanied by localized discomfort and referred pain patterns.

By employing a range of massage techniques and targeted pressure, trigger point massage seeks to alleviate tension, increase blood circulation, and promote musculoskeletal health as a whole.

Trigger point therapy is significant due to its capacity to alleviate a variety of ailments, such as chronic pain conditions, headaches, myofascial pain syndrome, and sports injuries.

Massage therapists have the ability to promote pain relief, enhanced range of motion, and improved overall well-being in their clients through the strategic targeting of trigger points.

Trigger point massage sessions are formulated through communication,

communication, and the application of a variety of tools and techniques. By incorporating trigger point massage alongside physical therapy, chiropractic care, acupuncture, and stress management techniques, a more holistic and comprehensive approach to musculoskeletal issues can be achieved.

The incorporation of self-care strategies, such as stretching, strengthening exercises, and stress management, is essential for preserving the advantageous effects of trigger point massage in the interim period.

Promoting client engagement in their health through the integration of these practices into their daily regimens cultivates a proactive and enduring approach to well-being.

Collaborative efforts among healthcare professionals, such as chiropractors, massage therapists, and physical therapists, among others, guarantee comprehensive and integrated care for individuals within the broader healthcare system.

This collaborative approach takes into account the complex and diverse aspects of health, encompassing psychological and lifestyle factors that influence overall well-being in addition to physical symptoms.

The continuous advancement of research and comprehension regarding trigger points holds the promise of further refining therapeutic approaches. Constantly evolving and adaptable, the domain of massage therapy, which encompasses trigger point massage, contributes to the continuous pursuit of efficacious resolutions for musculoskeletal concerns and the advancement of overall well-being.

THE END

www.ingramcontent.com/pod-product-compliance
Lightning Source LLC
Chambersburg PA
CBHW071602270726

48661CB00017B/358